How To Have The Best Pregnancy Ever

312 Great Tips For A Healthy Pregnancy

ADAM COLTON

Published by BizMove
www.bizmove.com

Table of Contents

---

1. Pregnancy Fact Sheet

Pregnancy lasts about 40 weeks, counting from the first day of your last normal period. The weeks are grouped into three trimesters.

First trimester (week 1–week 12)

During the first trimester your body undergoes many changes. Hormonal changes affect almost every organ system in your body. These changes can trigger symptoms even in the very first weeks of pregnancy. Your period stopping is a clear sign that you are pregnant. Other changes may include:

- Extreme tiredness
- Tender, swollen breasts. Your nipples might also stick out.
- Upset stomach with or without throwing up (morning sickness)
- Cravings or distaste for certain foods
- Mood swings
- Constipation (trouble having bowel movements)
- Need to pass urine more often
- Headache
- Heartburn

- Weight gain or loss

As your body changes, you might need to make changes to your daily routine, such as going to bed earlier or eating frequent, small meals. Fortunately, most of these discomforts will go away as your pregnancy progresses. And some women might not feel any discomfort at all! If you have been pregnant before, you might feel differently this time around. Just as each woman is different, so is each pregnancy.

Second trimester (week 13–week 28)

Most women find the second trimester of pregnancy easier than the first. But it is just as important to stay informed about your pregnancy during these months.

You might notice that symptoms like nausea and fatigue are going away. But other new, more noticeable changes to your body are now happening. Your abdomen will expand as the baby continues to grow. And before this trimester is over, you will feel your baby beginning to move!

As your body changes to make room for your growing baby, you may have:

- Body aches, such as back, abdomen, groin, or thigh pain
- Stretch marks on your abdomen, breasts, thighs, or buttocks
- Darkening of the skin around your nipples
- A line on the skin running from belly button to pubic hairline
- Patches of darker skin, usually over the cheeks, forehead, nose, or upper lip. Patches often match on both sides of the face. This is sometimes called the mask of pregnancy.
- Numb or tingling hands, called carpal tunnel syndrome
- Itching on the abdomen, palms, and soles of the feet. (Call your doctor if you have nausea, loss of appetite, vomiting, jaundice or fatigue combined with itching. These can be signs of a serious liver problem.)
- Swelling of the ankles, fingers, and face. (If you notice any sudden or extreme swelling or if you gain a lot of weight really quickly, call your doctor right away. This could be a sign of preeclampsia.)

Third trimester (week 29–week 40)

You're in the home stretch! Some of the same discomforts you had in your second trimester will continue. Plus, many women find breathing difficult and notice they have to go to the bathroom even more often. This is because the baby is getting bigger and it is putting more pressure on your organs. Don't worry, your baby is fine and these problems will lessen once you give birth.

Some new body changes you might notice in the third trimester include:

- Shortness of breath
- Heartburn
- Swelling of the ankles, fingers, and face. (If you notice any sudden or extreme swelling or if you gain a lot of weight really quickly, call your doctor right away. This could be a sign of preeclampsia.)
- Hemorrhoids
- Tender breasts, which may leak a watery pre-milk called colostrum (kuh-LOSS-struhm)
- Your belly button may stick out
- Trouble sleeping
- The baby "dropping", or moving lower in your abdomen
- Contractions, which can be a sign of real or false labor

As you near your due date, your cervix becomes thinner and softer (called effacing). This is a normal, natural process that helps the birth canal (vagina) to open during the birthing process. Your doctor will check your progress with a vaginal exam as you near your due date. Get excited — the final countdown has begun!

Your Developing Baby

First trimester (week 1-week 12)

At four to five weeks:

- Your baby's brain and spinal cord have begun to form.
- The heart begins to form.
- Arm and leg buds appear.
- Your baby is now an embryo and one-twenty-fifth inch long.

At eight weeks:

- All major organs and external body structures have begun to form.
- Your baby's heart beats with a regular rhythm.
- The arms and legs grow longer, and fingers and toes have begun to form.
- The sex organs begin to form.
- The eyes have moved forward on the face and eyelids have formed.
- The umbilical cord is clearly visible.
- At the end of eight weeks, your baby is a fetus and looks more like a human. Your baby is

nearly 1 inch long and weighs less than one-eighth ounce.

At 12 weeks:

- The nerves and muscles begin to work together. Your baby can make a fist.
- The external sex organs show if your baby is a boy or girl. A woman who has an ultrasound in the second trimester or later might be able to find out the baby's sex.
- Eyelids close to protect the developing eyes. They will not open again until the 28th week.
- Head growth has slowed, and your baby is much longer. Now, at about 3 inches long, your baby weighs almost an ounce.

Second trimester (week 13-week 28)

At 16 weeks:

- Muscle tissue and bone continue to form, creating a more complete skeleton.
- Skin begins to form. You can nearly see through it.
- Meconium (mih-KOH-nee-uhm) develops in your baby's intestinal tract. This will be your baby's first bowel movement.

- Your baby makes sucking motions with the mouth (sucking reflex).
- Your baby reaches a length of about 4 to 5 inches and weighs almost 3 ounces.

At 20 weeks:

- Your baby is more active. You might feel slight fluttering.
- Your baby is covered by fine, downy hair called lanugo (luh-NOO-goh) and a waxy coating called vernix. This protects the forming skin underneath.
- Eyebrows, eyelashes, fingernails, and toenails have formed. Your baby can even scratch itself.
- Your baby can hear and swallow.
- Now halfway through your pregnancy, your baby is about 6 inches long and weighs about 9 ounces.

At 24 weeks:

- Bone marrow begins to make blood cells.
- Taste buds form on your baby's tongue.
- Footprints and fingerprints have formed.
- Real hair begins to grow on your baby's head.
- The lungs are formed, but do not work.

- The hand and startle reflex develop.
- Your baby sleeps and wakes regularly.
- If your baby is a boy, his testicles begin to move from the abdomen into the scrotum. If your baby is a girl, her uterus and ovaries are in place, and a lifetime supply of eggs have formed in the ovaries.
- Your baby stores fat and has gained quite a bit of weight. Now at about 12 inches long, your baby weighs about 1½ pounds.

Third trimester (week 29-week 40)

At 32 weeks:

- Your baby's bones are fully formed, but still soft.
- Your baby's kicks and jabs are forceful.
- The eyes can open and close and sense changes in light.
- Lungs are not fully formed, but practice "breathing" movements occur.
- Your baby's body begins to store vital minerals, such as iron and calcium.
- Lanugo begins to fall off.
- Your baby is gaining weight quickly, about one-half pound a week. Now, your baby is about 15 to 17 inches long and weighs about 4 to 4½

pounds.

At 36 weeks:

- The protective waxy coating called vernix gets thicker.
- Body fat increases. Your baby is getting bigger and bigger and has less space to move around. Movements are less forceful, but you will feel stretches and wiggles.
- Your baby is about 16 to 19 inches long and weighs about 6 to 6½ pounds.

Weeks 37-40:

- By the end of 37 weeks, your baby is considered full term. Your baby's organs are ready to function on their own.
- As you near your due date, your baby may turn into a head-down position for birth. Most babies "present" head down.
- At birth, your baby may weigh somewhere between 6 pounds 2 ounces and 9 pounds 2 ounces and be 19 to 21 inches long. Most full-term babies fall within these ranges. But healthy babies come in many different sizes

2. 212 Great Tips For A Healthy Pregnancy

As beautiful and amazing as pregnancy is, there are a million things you need to know to make sure the two (or more) of you are healthy and to keep yourself as happy and as comfortable as possible. This book is going to provide you with some very useful advice you can put into practice immediately so read on!

1. Stop smoking immediately if you have found out that you are pregnant or if are trying to become pregnant. Smoking, as we all know, is incredibly dangerous for us but it becomes even more important to quit when we are trying to take care of a new life. Talk with your doctor immediately if you are having trouble quitting.

2. Go ahead and give in to your pregnancy cravings. Doctors aren't quite sure if cravings are a result of emotional changes or of nutritional deficits in your diet, but not getting the foods you crave can be stressful during a time when you don't need the added stress. Just be careful that your diet is healthy overall.

3. Take a childbirth class. Even for veteran parents, these educational sessions help expectant parents feel more confident about their situation and their abilities. The classes give parents a forum to ask questions and meet other families who are experiencing the same things they are. They also provide time for each couple to talk and spend time with one another.

4. Search your home for various chemicals that could cause harm to your unborn baby, and throw them out. Household items like cleaning solutions can have adverse effects on your pregnancy, so look for natural choices instead. Keep using natural cleaners when you bring your baby home.

5. Try not to wear clothing that is too tight when pregnant. This kind of clothing can actually cause your fetus to not get enough oxygen and make you uncomfortable. There are maternity jeans available for pregnant women. Also, when at home, try to wear sweatpants or pajama bottoms with a loose T-shirt.

6. Check into hiring a doula for your birth experiences and for the period right after. Doulas are mothers' helpers who are there to provide non-medical support during the labor process and the post

partum period. Having a doula will help you to have a shorter and more satisfying birth experience.

7. Pack a suitcase for your trip to the hospital early in your third trimester. It is better to be prepared in advance and to have the peace of mind of knowing you are ready. Ensure your camera, birthing plan, insurance cards, and all other essentials are packed.

8. You can read online stories about birthing to find out about the experiences of other women. These accounts are great, as they are firsthand experiences of the process. Choose from many different writings so you feel relaxed and at ease.

9. Call your doctor for anything that seems "off". You know your body better than anyone and if something doesn't feel right, then use that intuition and give your practitioner a call. They will decide if it's something they need to check out or not, but don't hesitate to seek help.

10. When you are pregnant, it is best to avoid or limit your caffeine intake. You can still have one cup of coffee in the morning, but no more than that. Try drinking decaff or half-caff if you can. Any caffeine that you drink will go straight to your baby and may have negative effects.

11.　　Take some precautions when traveling by plane. The second trimester is often noted as the best time to fly, because you are not experiencing morning sickness as often, and there is less risk of miscarriage. Always speak to your doctor first and make sure to drink a lot of water on the plane to stay hydrated. Get up and walk frequently to help avoid blood clots.

12.　　Remember that even the best-laid plans can change, including your birth plan. Try to be flexible about the details, and do not beat yourself up if everything does not happen exactly the way you envisioned it. Ultimately, you probably won't even care that your favorite song never played or that you never made it into the birthing pool.

13.　　During the throes of morning sickness, eat what you can stomach. Keeping a little bit of food in your tummy often helps to relieve nausea, and your baby will be just fine if you subsist solely on just a few types of foods for a few days. Eating enough calories is essential, so talk to your doctor if you are unable to keep anything down.

14.　　Don't be afraid to say no to anything you don't want to do. If you are too tired to keep a movie date, it's okay to skip it. You need to make sure that you are taking care of your body the best that you can, and everyone who is close to you will respect this.

15.   When trying to become pregnant, charting your menstrual cycles may help you pinpoint your ovulation date, which is the time you have the best chance of conceiving. There are a variety of online charting sites as well as smartphone apps that can help you keep track of your periods, mood fluctuations, symptoms and other information.

16.   Keep a journal while you are pregnant to record special memories and thoughts. This helps with the emotions you experience during pregnancy and also gives you a great keepsake to share with your child later in life. You can use your journal to capture milestones during the pregnancy as well as your thoughts and emotions through the process.

17.   Make sure you drink enough water when pregnant. Thirst causes you to eat more, so stay hydrated. Sometimes, people mistake thirst for hunger. If you've already eaten some food but still feel hungry, a full glass of water may be just what you need.

18.   Get prenatal vitamins from your doctor or over the counter and make sure you take them on a regular basis. A good prenatal vitamin will take care

of the needs of both you and your new baby. Make sure that your vitamin contains 0.4 mgs of folic acid for optimum brain development.

19.   Try taking your prenatal vitamins at night. These pills, while essential for the proper growth and development of your baby, can make some mothers feel nauseous. Taking them before you lay down or with food can help your body adjust to their effects. If you need to take them during the day, try chewing gum afterwards.

20.   Take a childbirth class. Even for veteran parents, these educational sessions help expectant parents feel more confident about their situation and their abilities. The classes give parents a forum to ask questions and meet other families who are experiencing the same things they are. They also provide time for each couple to talk and spend time with one another.

21.   Sleep whenever you get a chance to during your pregnancy. Difficulty sleeping is one of the biggest complaints women have while pregnant. As our bodies go through these massive changes, the ease of being able to get a full night's sleep decreases. Take naps when the opportunity presents itself.

22.   You should attend pregnancy classes as soon as you find out you are pregnant. These classes are designed to answer many of the questions that first time moms have. You should encourage the father to come with you so he can ask questions too.

23.   Drinking plenty of water is always a healthy choice and is essential during pregnancy. Many women experience dehydration which results in constipation and other difficulties related to it during pregnancy. So, make it your aim to drink forty-eight to sixty-four ounces per day and ward off the bad effects of dehydration.

24.   When preparing for sleep while pregnant, set up a bedtime routine. Include activities that will relax you. Some relaxing activities are, drinking warm milk, reading a book or having a warm shower. When you are relaxed, it will be easier for you to fall asleep. Be sure that you have your routine set up so that you allow yourself enough time for sleep.

25.   Pregnancy can be a stressful time for couples. So it is better to work on relationship issues as they arise than waiting until after the baby arrives. Counseling can help couples communicate better and strengthen your relationship, which in turn will help you both be better prepared to handle your new baby as partners.

26.   Be prepared for the hospital keep an old towel and a plastic bag in your car just in case your water breaks on the way to the hospital. Pack a robe for pacing the hospital halls, as well as nonskid slipper socks. Fill a small bag with electronics, such as an iPod for music and a still-photo and video camera. You will also need your insurance card, toiletries and a going home outfit for you and the baby. Staying prepared ensures this stressful time is easier, and keeps your emotions on a more even keel.

27.   Before you get pregnant, you and your partner should see a doctor for a physical exam. This allows you the opportunity to find out whether you should schedule any tests based on your medical history. In addition, it enables you to find out the answers to any questions you have in regard to your prospective pregnancy.

28.   Having to urinate frequently is something a lot of women experience during pregnancy. As the pregnancy progresses, the need to urinate will become more frequent as well. One tip to help with this is, when you urinate lean forward to ensure the bladder is completely empty, this could help to lessen your restroom trips.

29.   If you experience symptoms like blurred vision, pain in your right side, frequent headaches, very rapid weight gain, or cola-colored urine in the second half of your pregnancy, report them to your doctor immediately. You may be developing preeclampsia, a pregnancy-related condition that can be life-threatening. Your doctor may need to perform tests to check for protein in your urine, and your blood pressure will be closely monitored.

30.   It is always important to eat healhty, but when you are pregnant it is even more important. To keep your pregnancy running smooth and to have a healthy baby you should eat a variety of foods from each of the recommended food groups and make sure your diet is well balanced.

31.   Talk with your doctor about getting a DHA supplement during your pregnancy. DHA is a omega-3 fatty acid that is essential for proper development of the brain and eyes of your baby. Supplements are generally needed to ensure the proper amount of DHA. Fish is a strong source of DHA but women are generally told to stay away from most fish during pregnancy due to mercury levels so a supplement is generally your best bet.

32.   A healthy diet during pregnancy includes foods that are packed with nutrition to help your baby get

off to a great start. Include a variety of foods that provide the fiber, vitamins and minerals that will help your baby develop properly. Get rid of the nutritionally empty junk foods that use up your daily calorie intake with no benefit to your baby.

33.   You need to buy maternity bras and other clothing as you realize you need them. Maternity clothes will make you feel more comfortable, and you'll actually have clothes to wear outside your home. Don't be embarrassed to buy maternity clothing early. Be comfortable in your own skin and in what you are wearing.

34.   Don't be afraid to contact your doctor if you suffer any unusual symptoms during your pregnancy. These symptoms include stomach pain, cramping, vaginal bleeding, and especially a decreased level of fetal activity. It's difficult to tell if everything is okay from the outside, and you're better off asking your physician to check if something seems strange.

35.   Do not avoid sex when you are pregnant. Many women are under the assumption that sex can harm their unborn child, but this is not true. In fact, sex can be helpful. Women have high hormone levels when pregnant, and having sex can help relieve some of the stress that these hormones give them.

36.   Avoid any chemicals that could harm your baby. Many cleaning products have a strong smell and can be found in your home, your work and anywhere else you go. When you breath in these fumes, they can harm your child. Use products that are only made out of natural ingredients.

37.   It's crucial that you be tested for pregnancy the very moment you think you might be pregnant. Waiting too long to confirm a pregnancy can cause complications and stop you from getting all the necessary care.

38.   Take a childbirth class. Classes are offered in many doctors' offices and online. Topics covered include nutrition, exercise, relaxation, epidural anesthesia, pain relief in labor, preparing for labor and childbirth, as well as breastfeeding and baby care. Classes are generally offered once a week over a six to eight week period. Studies show that couples that attend regular childbirth classes are prepared and relaxed during childbirth.

39.   Eat healthy during pregnancy. Both the mother-to-be and her unborn fetus need a balanced diet. Because you are carrying a life within your body, you must take in more calories, about 300 more

each day. Remember to eat healthy food products like vegetables and fruit and drink lots of water.

40.   Keep yourself well hydrated. Your body takes on pounds of extra weight in the form of fluids and blood. You need to give your body what it needs to produce these things. What your body needs is water. Keep a water bottle with you everywhere you go and just refill it during the day.

41.   As you near the beginning of your 3rd trimester, you should go ahead and get a bag packed for the hospital. If you put this off, there is a chance you may have to go to the hospital without any of your belongings. You need a camera, insurance cards, birth plan, and batteries.

42.   One of the best things that you can do when you are pregnant, is to purchase books on pregnancy that will allow you to develop a structure for what to expect in the upcoming months. This will assure that there are no surprises so that you are prepared when the time comes to give birth.

43.   Make sure you can say no to food. You need to take in more calories when you are pregnant, but you don't need to eat at all times. Politely decline food if you are no longer hungry.

44.   Start a journal or a pregnancy blog and post this online. Sharing your experiences can be very beneficial as the people who are reading your blog can offer you advice that is unique to your stage in pregnancy. Also, this will give you documentation of how you felt during each step of the process.

45.   When choosing items for your hospital bag, include some of your creature comforts to make your stay more pleasant. Items like your favorite lip balm or soft socks are good to have, and don't forget to pack a few toiletries, snacks and a change of clothes for your partner if he or she will be staying with you.

46.   Do not give up exercising when you are pregnant, unless you have a medically necessary reason to do so. Low-impact exercises, such as swimming or walking, are great ways to help your muscles stay strong. Exercising can also help make your labor easier.

47.   Make sure that you understand which pregnancy-related expenses your health insurance does, and does not cover, including prenatal visits, tests, and ultrasounds. Having an idea of what you will owe ahead of time - including your deductible - can reduce the shock when the bills do start rolling in.

48.   Browse consignment or resale shops for great deals on maternity clothing. Since maternity clothes are worn for a relatively short period of time, it isn't uncommon to find like-new tops, pants, dresses and outerwear for a fraction of retail price. When you are finished with them, you can resell them yourself or pass them on to a friend or family member.

49.   You should eat enough while pregnant. Being pregnant requires your body to consume about 300 more calories than normal. If you are also exercising, it will increase your calorie needs even more. Your body knows what it wants, if you are hungry, you need to eat, just make sure to make good food choices.

50.   Before you get pregnant you should read a book about being pregnant. This way you will know what to expect during pregnancy. Pregnancy books can also teach you many different things you may not have known about being pregnant. You will learn new things along with terminology about pregnancy.

51.   Try taking your prenatal vitamins at night. These pills, while essential for the proper growth and development of your baby, can make some mothers feel nauseous. Taking them before you lay down or

with food can help your body adjust to their effects. If you need to take them during the day, try chewing gum afterwards.

52.   Before giving birth, visit the hospital first. Meet the nursing staff and get a tour. Doing this will help you know what to expect and bring you piece of mind. Bring the father along too since they will communicate with the staff when you're in labor.

53.   Drinking plenty of water is always a healthy choice and is essential during pregnancy. Many women experience dehydration which results in constipation and other difficulties related to it during pregnancy. So, make it your aim to drink forty-eight to sixty-four ounces per day and ward off the bad effects of dehydration.

54.   When you are pregnant and your stomach finally starts expanding go buy yourself some comfortable maternity clothes. Your going to be pregnant for the next several months, so you might as well be comfortable. This also makes sure that you don't have to keep buying new clothes as you continuously expand.

55.   When you are in the later stages of pregnancy, especially in your third trimester, try not to travel too much. Some women think that because their

due date is a month away, they will not go into labor on the train or plane, only to find themselves delivering their child with no medical assistance.

56.   Eat plenty of fruit during your pregnancy. Many women get a boost of energy during the day from caffeine products; since these are not recommended during pregnancy, try fruit instead. People who consume bananas and apples, often notice an increase in their energy levels. This comes from the natural sugars that these fruits contain.

57.   It is advised that pregnant women wear sports bras. A sports bra will give additional support for your breasts and will help with aches and pains in them as well. Furthermore, do not wear underwear that is too tight around your waist. It can cut off oxygen to the baby and also cause discomfort for you.

58.   Make sure to keep the windows wide open if you are doing any decorating with paint or glue during your pregnancy. Paint and wallpaper projects can release harmful fumes into your nursery. Keeping the windows open will dissipate the fumes and help you to avoid any harmful effect on your baby.

59.	Pregnancy can be a stressful time for couples. So it is better to work on relationship issues as they arise than waiting until after the baby arrives. Counseling can help couples communicate better and strengthen your relationship, which in turn will help you both be better prepared to handle your new baby as partners.

60.	Being pregnant can be exhausting because you are doing everything for two. One tip is to slow down and take a short nap whenever you can. It will be good for you and your baby, just to forget about everything and take a power nap to try to refresh yourself and take a break.

61.	Birth plans are a great way to get organized during your pregnancy. Right down what would make you comfortable when giving birth. This may mean how you want the lighting or what music you want to hear. It can be complex or simple; it's up to you.

62.	Rest and relaxation are especially important during pregnancy to make sure that your baby is not stressed while slowly growing and developing inside. Take time for a break every day with soft lights and music to sooth away the stress of your every day routine. Even just a few minutes can make a big difference.

63.   Avoid emptying the kitty's cat box during pregnancy. If there is no way to avoid this chore wear gloves and a mask. There is a small chance of contacting a parasitic infection called toxoplasmosis from cat stool. Since it takes 48 hours for the spores to become infectious, the litter box should also be changed everyday. It is also a good idea to wear gloves when gardening, since neighborhood cats often defecate in flowerbeds.

64.   To avoid pain while sleeping, do a set of stretches prior to getting in bed. Cramping in the legs, especially the calves, is a very common complaint for pregnant women. This is due to the extra weight and strain on the leg muscles. You can help prevent leg cramping during the night with a regular stretching routine to relax your leg muscles before bed. This is a great way to relax your body and rest soundly.

65.   You need to exercise while you are pregnant. It is important to keep your body as healthy and fit as you can even during pregnancy. A pregnant woman who has kept herself in shape will have an easier time during delivery and may even experience fewer contractions during labor, which is what every woman really wants.

66.   Eat plenty of foods that contain choline during your pregnancy. Choline is crucial in a developing fetus' brain development. If you do not get enough choline it can lead to damaged brain development in your growing baby. You can find choline in foods like eggs, beef, and dairy products.

67.   It is not too early to start with a prenatal vitamin, even before you conceive. Your baby will start growing their neural cord, which will then turn into the baby's brain and spinal cord, while you are in your first trimester of being pregnant. Make sure you are getting the right amount of calcium, iron and folic acid because it is essential, even at the start of your conception adventure.

68.   Don't be afraid to contact your doctor if you suffer any unusual symptoms during your pregnancy. These symptoms include stomach pain, cramping, vaginal bleeding, and especially a decreased level of fetal activity. It's difficult to tell if everything is okay from the outside, and you're better off asking your physician to check if something seems strange.

69.   Do not feel required to announce your pregnancy to everyone as soon as you know. All women have their own comfort zone regarding when they want to tell everyone. Some women wait

until they have reached the end of the first trimester and the highest risk of miscarriage is over. Listen to your heart and share the news when you are ready to.

70.   It is important for pregnant women to avoid eating certain fish, like shark, swordfish, and tilefish. These fish contain high levels of mercury, which can cause health problems for your baby. There are some seafood that is safe for pregnant women to eat including canned tuna, pollack, salmon, catfish, and shrimp.

71.   When you are pregnant, one of the things that you will want to stop as soon as possible is smoking. Smoking can cause birth defects for your baby, so stopping immediately will limit this risk. Join support groups to increase the willpower that you will need to stop this unhealthy habit. You must also insist that people who smoke do not do so in the same room as you.

72.   One of the best things that you can do when you are pregnant, is to purchase books on pregnancy that will allow you to develop a structure for what to expect in the upcoming months. This will assure that there are no surprises so that you are prepared when the time comes to give birth.

73.   When you are pregnant, it is best to avoid or limit your caffeine intake. You can still have one cup of coffee in the morning, but no more than that. Try drinking decaff or half-caff if you can. Any caffeine that you drink will go straight to your baby and may have negative effects.

74.   When you are pregnant it may be beneficial to find a support group. Being a pregnant woman is certainly not easy. Between the emotions, and the physical sicknesses that accompany it , it can be quite a trying time. Find friends, and others that have been through it that can help support you till delivery day.

75.   In late pregnancy, you should avoid sleeping on your back, if possible. If you find it difficult to stay off your back, try propping a pillow behind you so that you are not able to roll into a completely flat position. There is no need to panic if you do occasionally wake up on your back; generally, you will feel very uncomfortable in that position before causing any harm to yourself or your baby.

76.   Grab some rubber bands if you want to keep wearing your favorite jeans through your pregnancy. A neat trick is to take a heavy rubber band and put it through the buttonhole in your jeans. Attach both ends of the rubber band to the button and voila,

extra space. Wear longer shirts over the jeans to hide the rubber band.

77.   Don't leave the house without a change of clothes and a fresh pair of underwear. Pregnancy leaves us with a lot less control over our bodies and accidents can happen. It is better to act like a boy scout and be prepared than have to run home in the middle of the day because we were caught off guard.

78.   Talk to your baby. Studies have shown that babies do react to touch from ten weeks in the pregnancy. At later stages they can react to light, your voice as well as other sounds. This will bond you and your baby for life, and while they won't remember any of this, it will definitely help.

79.   Staying organized with lists and priorities during your pregnancy can relieve a lot of the stress. Don't forget that you can ask friends and family to help with things on your list. Sometimes, you might be able to drop unimportant tasks from your list, also.

80.   It is always important to eat healhty, but when you are pregnant it is even more important. To keep your pregnancy running smooth and to have a healthy baby you should eat a variety of foods from

each of the recommended food groups and make sure your diet is well balanced.

81. Make sure that the extra calories you consume during pregnancy are nutritious ones. Try having a yogurt and fruit as a morning snack, and a sandwich with 2 ounces of chicken to add your calories without overeating. Do go ahead and splurge on a treat every once in a while.

82. When pregnant, make sure you are 100% comfortable with the doctor or OB/GYN who will be delivering your child. If you are not, search for another one until you are. Ask questions when you need an answer, there is nothing your doctor has not heard before. And make sure you check out the delivery facilities prior to the birth so you are completely comfortable with where your child will be born. All these things will ensure that your pregnancy is calmer and less stressful.

83. Don't stop using a seat belt in your car while driving or riding as a passenger. The danger to your baby from the seat belt is much less than the danger from you being loose in the car in the event of a crash. Make sure the belt is as low on your hips as possible, preferably underneath your belly.

84.   When riding in a car that has air bags, have the seat pushed back as far as possible from the dashboard. The closer you are to the dash, the closer you are to the airbags. Airbags can be dangerous to an unborn baby, though turning them off is more dangerous to you, so simply sit further away to balance these risks.

85.   Don't travel in the later stages of pregnancy, without discussing it with your doctor, first. Ensure that your medical records are traveling with you, just in case there are any issues.

86.   If you are a smoker, now is the time to quit. Many programs are around to help you do this. Smoking can lead to having a premature baby. It can also cause your baby to be underweight. Babies need to start out with a strong start, in order to be prepared to handle this world.

87.   If you get a headache when you are pregnant, make sure to stay away from aspirin. Aspirin has been proven to cause harm in both an expectant mother and baby. It is best to ask your doctor what medications are safe for you to use. Also, try relieving head pressure by using a cool compress.

88.   Take a childbirth class. Even for veteran parents, these educational sessions help expectant

parents feel more confident about their situation and their abilities. The classes give parents a forum to ask questions and meet other families who are experiencing the same things they are. They also provide time for each couple to talk and spend time with one another.

89.   For pregnant women, make sure that you stretch your legs, before going to sleep every night. This is because many pregnant women get intense muscle cramps while they are sleeping, which could be easily prevented, if they stretch. Spend about 5 minutes flexing all of your muscles, before even climbing into bed.

90.   If you are pregnant and feeling constant cravings, sometimes it may not be wise to fulfill them all. Your child has nutritional needs as well. Gorging yourself on your cravings may only satisfy those cravings and not the nutritional needs of your unborn child. For this reason, make sure you eat a well-balanced to meet both of your needs.

91.   If you are pregnant, make sure to elevate your feet when you are resting at home. This helps to prevent swelling and take away the pains that pregnancy causes in the feet. Lay on your back, place at least 2 pillows underneath your feet and then put your feet up.

92.   To keep wearing your own pants tie a rubber band on your button and loop through your button hole. With a long shirt or an elastic maternity band to cover the top of your pants, no one can tell that they are technically unbuttoned. This will enable you to avoid wasting money on maternity pants too early.

93.   Avoid plastic containers that have BPA during your pregnancy. BPA acts like estrogen in the body and can have an adverse effect on babies. The BPA can have a feminizing affect on the fetus that you want to avoid. Switch out your plastics for glass and stainless steel to avoid the risk.

94.   Make sure the prescription drugs you are taking are not dangerous to the health of your baby. Every prescription drug on the market has a "pregnancy class" that tells you whether the drug is safe to take during pregnancy. If you are taking a drug that is unsafe for pregnant women, ask your doctor about alternatives. Most drugs have one or more.

95.   Before you begin trying to conceive a baby, visit your doctor and check to be sure your vaccinations are updated. In particular, you want to make sure that you have the rubella and varicella vaccines. Exposure to these two diseases could be

detrimental to your pregnancy if you haven't already been protected.

96.   Being pregnant can be exhausting because you are doing everything for two. One tip is to slow down and take a short nap whenever you can. It will be good for you and your baby, just to forget about everything and take a power nap to try to refresh yourself and take a break.

97.   Most pregnant women suffer from morning sickness. There are many options available that can help women feel better during down periods of morning sickness. Eat meals that are smaller and eat more frequently, as opposed to staying hungry. You need to stay hydrated, be certain to take in alot of fluids during the day. Never take prenatal vitamins on an empty stomach. Instead, take them with food and plenty of water. You should stay away from certain foods that do not make you feel good. Getting enough rest during the day and adequate sleep at night can make a big difference in how well you feel.

98.   Do not do too much when you are exercising while you are pregnant. This will ensure that you do not overextend yourself. It is very important to not hurt yourself when you are exercising when

pregnant. It can not only make your pregnancy tougher on you but also on the baby, as well.

99.	Make sure you are getting plenty of sleep each night. You need around 8 hours. Getting the right amount of sleep will help you to feel good, and it will also help your fetus to grow. During pregnancy many people feel very tired, and it is important to give your body what it needs.

100.	Do not avoid sex when you are pregnant. Many women are under the assumption that sex can harm their unborn child, but this is not true. In fact, sex can be helpful. Women have high hormone levels when pregnant, and having sex can help relieve some of the stress that these hormones give them.

101.	Pregnancy is both a positive and challenging thing to have happen in your life. The positive part about it is bringing something new into the world. The challenging parts are dealing with not only physical changes, but mental as well. You may experience different moods and things you're not used to and a doctor will very much be willing to help and a valuable ally in your new adventure.

102.	Avoid any chemicals that could harm your baby. Many cleaning products have a strong smell and can be found in your home, your work and anywhere else you go. When you breath in these fumes, they can harm your child. Use products that are only made out of natural ingredients.

103.   Pack your bags early. Don't wait until you are 37 weeks or later to finally pack your bag for the hospital. Obviously you want your baby to reach full gestation, but you never know when something is going to happen. Having your bag packed will give you peace of mind in case there is an unexpected event.

104.   Consider hiring a doula. Dolulas are trained professionals that help coach a woman during labor. Their support can be both moral and physical. They help your birthing experience to be a good one.

105.   Try exercise classes that are designed for pregnant women. Staying active is very important during pregnancy but it is also important that you exercise safely. Going to a class that is specifically created for pregnancy means that you will gain all the benefits of the exercise without doing any damage to your growing baby.

106.   Once the third trimester rolls around, you should ensure your hospital bag is packed and ready to go. It is better to be prepared in advance and to have the peace of mind of knowing you are ready.

You should have your birth plan, a camera, memory cards, extra battery and insurance cards with you.

107.   Be prepared to lose a few extra strands of hair in the postpartum period. Many women are not aware that this is common and are alarmed when it occurs. The extra shedding is likely due to hormonal changes and should stop within a couple of months. If it continues for a long time or you are concerned, ask your doctor to check your thyroid levels.

108.   Wear plenty of sunscreen while you are pregnant. You are more likely to become sunburned and get dark spots on your face during pregnancy. Try to apply a lotion with an SPF of at least 30 and stay away from tanning beds. Wear a hat and sunglasses for extra protection.

109.   During the throes of morning sickness, eat what you can stomach. Keeping a little bit of food in your tummy often helps to relieve nausea, and your baby will be just fine if you subsist solely on just a few types of foods for a few days. Eating enough calories is essential, so talk to your doctor if you are unable to keep anything down.

110.   Shortness of breath is common as women progress in their pregnancy. The baby grows and compresses the diaphragm, so there is less room to

breathe. To help with this do some pelvic tilts and light stretching. Also, sleeping sitting up works well for some women as it relieves some of the pressure and allows them to breathe more freely.

111.   Avoid using products to cleanse your vagina during your pregnancy. These products may cause health problems in your baby. If you have an unusual odor, talk with your obstetrician about the possible cause and solution.

112.   When you are pregnant, you will want to let someone else clean out your precious cat's litter box. This is because there is a parasite in cat feces that causes toxoplasmosis. This parasite is also found in rare or raw meat. This can lead to serious illness, miscarriage, premature birth or even worse. So cook your meat well, and let your loved one clean the litter box.

113.   Make sure to schedule some last minute pampering before the baby is born. Get your hair cut and your nails done. After the baby is born it may be a long long time before you will be able to do that again. If you do get a chance to do it you will be anxious to get back as soon as possible. Take advantage of the time you have and enjoy it before the baby is born.

114. When you are pregnant, you may experience heartburn. The hormone, progesterone, is released as soon as you become pregnant and may cause pregnancy heartburn. Naturally, avoiding spicy, fatty and acidic foods is helpful. This is especially true just before bedtime. Keep you head elevated while sleeping as an extra precaution. Talk to your doctor if it becomes unbearable.

115. A few weeks before the baby is due start preparing some extra meals, or double or triple your recipes and freeze the extra. When the baby comes and you are adjusting to your new routine it will be nice to have those ready-made meals that you can just pop in the oven.

116. Sleep as much as you want while you are pregnant. Sleep is in short supply for the parents of newborns. Also, while pregnant, your baby is eating up much of your available energy. Don't be afraid to sleep in, go to bed early, or nap when you want to. You won't be able to later!

117. Don't stop using a seat belt in your car while driving or riding as a passenger. The danger to your baby from the seat belt is much less than the danger from you being loose in the car in the event of a crash. Make sure the belt is as low on your hips as possible, preferably underneath your belly.

118.   Start taking a prenatal vitamin while you are
       trying to conceive, or as soon as you first find out
       about that surprise pregnancy. There are special
       nutrients that are needed by your baby for proper
       development. The sooner you start taking prenatal
       vitamins, the better chance your baby has of getting
       the nutrients he or she needs.

119.   Get prenatal vitamins from your doctor or over
       the counter and make sure you take them on a
       regular basis. A good prenatal vitamin will take care
       of the needs of both you and your new baby. Make
       sure that your vitamin contains 0.4 mgs of folic acid
       for optimum brain development.

120.   Wear sunscreen while pregnant, even if you
       didn't really require it before. You should also avoid
       using a tanning bed. During pregnancy, your skin
       will become more sensitive, so avoid anything that
       is too harsh. Check the label of your sunscreen and
       other skin care products to make sure it does not
       contain harmful chemicals.

121.   When you need to lift something while
       pregnant, do not be afraid to ask someone to help
       you with it. Heavy lifting is especially hard on your
       pregnant body, and if you strain too much you can
       hurt your baby or even cause early labor. Always get

someone to help lift objects, never overexert yourself.

122.   Try babysitting a friend's baby to get more comfortable with caring for a newborn. Having some hands on experience will help you feel more comfortable with the impending birth of your new baby. Don't take off more than you can chew though as you get farther along in your pregnancy.

123.   Invest in comfortable shoes when you're pregnant, as it will definitely help you. You are walking around with a lot of extra weight that your body is not use to, and it will take its tole on your feet. You will find they will start to swell, and you need shoes that are non-restrictive to battle this.

124.   During your last trimester of pregnancy, your body will go through many changes. That's no surprise, but one thing that even your doctor might forget to mention is that, as your baby grows, your belly button can be pushed outwards so that it protrudes like a miniature bumper guard on your stomach.

125.   Be sure to see your doctor before becoming pregnant. Not only does this help establish a healthy start to your prenatal care should you become pregnant, it also allows your doctor to check for any

conditions that might require special care, or worse, discover conditions that would make pregnancy dangerous.

126.   Realize that "morning" sickness can happen at any time of the day and check with your doctor if it seems really bad. Most new parents are only affected by morning sickness during the first trimester of pregnancy. It is usually one of the first signs that a women picks up on to signify that she may be pregnant. If it is keeping you from being able to keep down any food, see your doctor for ideas on how to help.

127.   If you have decided how to have your baby, maybe natural childbirth, or caesarian section, you should write a birth plan. The birth plan will detail all of your expectations for delivery and should be shared with your doctors. Having this plan will calm your anxiety as your delivery date approaches.

128.   Late pregnancy back pain is a reality that most women have to deal with. In order to minimize the pain, you need to have a massage to help loosen the muscles. If massage is not an option, pelvic tilts or hot compresses will also work very well to relieve some of the pressure.

129.   You can learn a great deal during your pregnancy to prepare for the birth of your child by reading about the birth experiences of others. Reading the stories that others share, and watching videos that they have posted online can give you valuable information about the wonders of birth, as well as the challenges.

130.   Keep your calcium intake high during pregnancy. Your baby needs the calcium for its development. If you are not giving your body enough calcium, it will leech the calcium it needs from your bones. This will put you at risk for osteoporosis down the road. So make sure you drink that glass of milk in the mornings.

131.   If you often experience mood swings while you are pregnant, yoga or meditation may help. Both can really help you relax in a natural way. You could ask a stressed partner to accompany you to yoga or meditation classes, as well.

132.   If you get diagnosed with gestational diabetes or some other issue that pertains to strictly the time when you are pregnant, know that this is just a temporary thing. It will help you get through the days of your pregnancy knowing that as soon as you are holding your baby you will know that it was all worth it.

133. Before you get pregnant, you should see your doctor. This way your doctor can recommend safe practices for you to have while trying to conceive. They can recommend foods you should eat and things you should avoid. They can also let you know things that can make it harder to conceive.

134. When riding in a car that has air bags, have the seat pushed back as far as possible from the dashboard. The closer you are to the dash, the closer you are to the airbags. Airbags can be dangerous to an unborn baby, though turning them off is more dangerous to you, so simply sit further away to balance these risks.

135. Write a birth plan early in your pregnancy. Keep a list of the things you absolutely want to have happen, like the presence of an older sibling, and things you absolutely don't want unless it begins to affect the safety of the baby. If you have these things written down ahead of time, you can discuss them with your birth team and make sure they happen.

136. To give your baby a healthy start in life, make sure you change to a healthy diet while pregnant. If you had a habit of consuming a lot of fatty foods before becoming pregnant, you need to change your

lifestyle quickly. Eat more vegetables, fruits and lean protein.

137.   Have your significant other make healthy changes in their life as well. As you make all these big changes in your eating habits and activities, having someone to lean on will be a big advantage. If you do it together, it will help you both keep on track with these changes.

138.   Take your iron pills. Many pregnant women will get anemia at some point during their pregnancy. Your body needs a lot of iron reserves for the birth and after when you are breastfeeding. Ask your doctor early about taking an iron supplement to keep your levels high and prevent anemia in the first place.

139.   Lower your intake of vitamin A when pregnant. Vitamin A can sometimes damage your developing baby. Don't eat foods with this vitamin. You should avoid foods like egg yolks, mangoes, liver, and mozzarella cheese. You can eat a little, but do not consume vitamin A in bulk.

140.   A great thing that you can do, in order to have a healthy pregnancy, is to educate yourself. This is very important, especially to women who are pregnant for the first time. This can be done by

reading books related to pregnancy and in the long run, will help not only when laboring but also, when preparing for it.

141.   If you are working at a desk job during your pregnancy, you will need to make sure that you have lots of times during the day that you can get up and walk. Sitting down will put extra stress on your tailbone and hips, which are already absorbing a great deal more weight. Taking walks and moving around frequently will help keep this from becoming a problem.

142.   Eat five or six well-balanced meals every day. This will help you to get all the nutrition that you need, as well as the calories. You should not be eating junk food all day. There is no nutritional value in that, and the only thing it will do for you is put on extra pounds.

143.   Avoid pesticides by eating locally grown organic foods. We don't know how much effect these pesticides can have on a fetus but it is better to be safe than sorry. If not buying organic, stick with items with heavy peels like oranges as they are likely to be less contaminated.

144.   If you plan on painting your baby's nursery while you are pregnant, try to choose paints labeled

as "no-VOC" or "low-VOC." This distinction means the paints will release fewer volatile organic compounds -- like formaldehyde -- into the air, which is better for both your family's health and for the environment.

145.   In order to find the best nutrition for you and your baby during pregnancy, become a label reader. There are many extra chemicals and ingredients that may not be best for your growing baby and reading labels is the way to keep them out of your diet. It just takes a minute to protect your baby.

146.   It seems like when you are pregnant you just get used to looking down at swollen feet and ankles. One tip for instant relief is to soak them in cold water, you will be amazed at how quickly this works and how great you will feel. Just soak them for about twenty minutes and you will notice an immediate change.

147.   Leg cramps are a common occurrence during pregnancy and can be annoying. To minimize the cramping you should exercise, make sure you get enough calcium each day, and finally you do a few light stretches just before going to bed. That should help you avoid leg cramps while you sleep.

148.   To help ease nausea and vomiting during pregnancy, you should snack often and drink plenty of water or other liquids. It can also help to avoid situations that trigger your feelings of nausea when you can. If the smell of a certain food cooking brings on the feeling, save that recipe for after the baby is born.

149.   If you've never used sunscreen, you may want to start using it during your pregnancy. Also, make sure to always avoid tanning beds. Your skin may be more sensitive while you are pregnant, making sunburn or sunspots more likely. Make sure that any sunscreen you use is safe for your unborn baby.

150.   Avoid using over the counter medicines for digestive issues like heartburn, upset stomach and constipation. The more medicines we keep out of our bodies during pregnancy the better. Ginger tea, acupuncture and peppermint oils have all been shown to help with pregnancy stomach issues.

151.   Cease changing cat litter if you're pregnant. Toxoplasmosis is a risk for pregnant women that you can contract from contact with cat litter. Cats are a host for the toxoplasmosis life cycle, and if the infection is passed to the fetus, the consequences in pregnant women can lead to miscarriage, birth abnormalities and stillbirth.

152.   Increase your intake of cereals, asparagus, lentils, oranges and orange juice. These foods are all rich in folic acid, which helps the development of the baby's neural cord and creates red blood cells for your unborn child. It is ideal to begin consuming these foods even before you start trying to conceive.

153.   Tell your doctor if you start to experience a high level of vaginal discharge. You can have a vaginal infection, this is common when you are pregnant. If you do not fix the problem, you can have serious health issues for your baby.

154.   Start a journal or a pregnancy blog and post this online. Sharing your experiences can be very beneficial as the people who are reading your blog can offer you advice that is unique to your stage in pregnancy. Also, this will give you documentation of how you felt during each step of the process.

155.   Allow yourself to indulge in some of your cravings. You want to try and maintain a healthy diet during pregnancy, but it is okay to eat some unhealthy foods in moderation. Make sure to stay away from brie and feta cheese, herbal teas and raw sprouts, which could all negatively affect your baby's health.

156.   Stop taking any birth control the very minute you find out that you are pregnant. If it has failed to prevent your pregnancy, you do not want to continue it while you are pregnant. It has many negative health effects on the baby and the sooner you stop, the better the chances that the baby will be fine.

157.   One way to help to get rid of the back pain that sometimes occurs in late pregnancy is to practice pelvic tilts. Continuing to exercise in this way will not only help with the pain, it may also move your baby into a good birth position at the same time.

158.   Find out what blood type you and your partner have. If you have incompatible blood types, there is a possibility that you could also be incompatible with your baby's blood type. This can lead to a condition called anemia, which causes complications during the pregnancy and birth of your child.

159.   Get plenty of pregnancy before, during and after your pregnancy! Exercise lowers your rick of miscarrying, makes your pregnancy easier, results in fewer complications during labor and can even make your labor shorter. Regardless of whether you are already pregnant or you are trying to get

pregnant, exercise makes an easier time of the whole experience.

160.   To help prevent substantial weight gain during pregnancy, make sure that you eat breakfast. Missing this early meal often means that you will eat more later in the day, contributing to additional weight gain. In addition, your unborn child needs the nutrients from breakfast since a substantial amount of time has passed since your last meal.

161.   Stay active during your pregnancy to improve your health and make childbirth easier. Walking and swimming are great exercises even late in pregnancy. Staying active can keep your mood positive and make the process of giving birth less traumatic physically. If you have concerns about exercise, talk with your doctor to determine what activities are appropriate for you.

162.   You should eat enough while pregnant. Being pregnant requires your body to consume about 300 more calories than normal. If you are also exercising, it will increase your calorie needs even more. Your body knows what it wants, if you are hungry, you need to eat, just make sure to make good food choices.

163.   During pregnancy, you are more prone to injuries so it is best to avoid unstable ground and rocky terrain. Your body is readying itself for birth and is releasing a hormone in the body called relaxin. This hormone helps to loosen your pelvis so the baby can pass through easily. This makes your joints looser, and makes it easier for you to get hurt.

164.   Invest in a body pillow to help you sleep during pregnancy. Due to the changes in the body, it can be difficult to find a comfortable sleep position. A body pillow allows you to give your legs or back extra support and is flexible enough to be rearranged easily to find a new position.

165.   If you want to have a healthy pregnancy, it is best to see your doctor before you even decide to become pregnant. This is because you want to be sure that your body is ready for conception, pregnancy and delivery. After all, you want to be sure you and your baby will both be healthy.

166.   Start taking a prenatal vitamin while you are trying to conceive, or as soon as you first find out about that surprise pregnancy. There are special nutrients that are needed by your baby for proper development. The sooner you start taking prenatal

vitamins, the better chance your baby has of getting the nutrients he or she needs.

167.   Before you get pregnant you should read a book about being pregnant. This way you will know what to expect during pregnancy. Pregnancy books can also teach you many different things you may not have known about being pregnant. You will learn new things along with terminology about pregnancy.

168.   Don't be afraid to contact your doctor if you suffer any unusual symptoms during your pregnancy. These symptoms include stomach pain, cramping, vaginal bleeding, and especially a decreased level of fetal activity. It's difficult to tell if everything is okay from the outside, and you're better off asking your physician to check if something seems strange.

169.   Take a childbirth class. Even for veteran parents, these educational sessions help expectant parents feel more confident about their situation and their abilities. The classes give parents a forum to ask questions and meet other families who are experiencing the same things they are. They also provide time for each couple to talk and spend time with one another.

170.   One of the best things that women can do in order to achieve a healthy pregnancy is to exercise. This will not only help you to stay in shape during pregnancy, but it also lowers the risk of miscarriage. It has been proven that exercise reduces labor complications and length.

171.   During your pregnancy, ask others to help you lift things, instead of trying to do it yourself. Lifting heavy things can cause miscarriages or stress on your baby, not to mention that it can cause back strains. So, even though you think the weight is manageable to you, you should still have someone lift and carry heavy items for you.

172.   Read a pregnancy book. They provide expectant parents with a wealth of information on what to expect both during the pregnancy and after the baby is born. They give new parents piece of mind by helping them plan, and they answer questions that they may not want to ask their friends or family members.

173.   When you are going through pregnancy, be certain to get sufficient levels of protein intake. Protein is a very important nutrient that is good for you, and one your baby needs to grow healthy. There are many high protein foods you can choose from including pumpkin seeds, nuts, eggs,

hamburger meat, legumes, chicken, tofu, and sunflower seeds.

174.   Bland and low tasting food, such as crackers, are an ideal foodstuff to eat during the day while pregnant. When your stomach contains bland foods, the nausea should be lessened. Also, remember to avoid eating greasy, high acid foods. These foods will cause heartburn and increased nausea.

175.   Take a child birthing class. These classes will help you near the end of your pregnancy. They will teach you exactly what to expect, and your partner should go along to. You will probably watch a movie of someone giving birth, learn a lot of new breathing exercises, and probably meet some new friends too.

176.   Sleeping will become harder for you during your pregnancy. During the third trimester, sleep on your left side, this will provide you with the best blood flow to your fetus, uterus and kidneys. Remember, not to lay on your back.

177.   During your pregnancy it is important to get a full nights rest. Stress can be a major cause of not being able to sleep. If you are feeling stressed, find someone that you can talk to about the problems

that you are having. Pregnancy can be a stressful thing and you should always talk about the things that are causing you stress.

178.   It's really important to remember to make time for yourself. When you finally give birth, life will become much more complicated than right now, and you are going to have much less time to pamper yourself. You should take care of yourself by doing things you enjoy. Whether you'd prefer to do solitary activities, like engaging in a favorite hobby or do things with friends, participate in your favorite activities as much as possible while you still can. You will feel much better, and so will your unborn child.

179.   Be prepared for the hospital keep an old towel and a plastic bag in your car just in case your water breaks on the way to the hospital. Pack a robe for pacing the hospital halls, as well as nonskid slipper socks. Fill a small bag with electronics, such as an iPod for music and a still-photo and video camera. You will also need your insurance card, toiletries and a going home outfit for you and the baby. Staying prepared ensures this stressful time is easier, and keeps your emotions on a more even keel.

180.   Belching, gas, and heartburn are all side effects of being pregnant. To help deal with these types of

issues during your pregnancy, you should stay upright after you eat, stay away from offending foods, and drink a glass of milk with honey; these are all ways to help you minimize some of the gas and heartburn.

181.   It is important that pregnant women make a labor plan before the big day comes. This is because when a woman is in labor, she may not be able to make decisions like she normally does. Make sure you have a bag packed, pick out who you want in the room when you give birth and make a list of phone numbers so your spouse or other family members can call your loved ones when the baby is born.

182.   If you are seeing a doctor for anything, you need to tell them that you are pregnant. Some of the tests that they perform at the doctors office can be harmful to a pregnant women, and they will skip these for you. Even if there is only a small chance you could be pregnant, you need to speak up.

183.   Educate yourself on when you need to pick up the phone and call your doctor when dealing with premature labor. You will, hopefully, not ever use this information. Still, it is good to be prepared just in case. The sooner you respond and the quicker

you take the proper steps, the better your outcome will be.

184.   If you are pregnant and concerned with unsightly stretch marks post-pregnancy, it would be wise to invest in some cocoa butter. It has been shown that regular use of cocoa butter during and after pregnancy reduce and/or eliminate the appearance of unsightly stretch marks. So go get yourself a tub of it today!

185.   When pregnant, avoid drinking excessively before you go to sleep. It is important to drink enough fluids during the day to keep you hydrated. However, you should stop drinking about two hours before going to sleep. This will help you avoid frequent trips to the bathroom when you should be sleeping.

186.   Talk to any friend who has given birth to learn some tricks and tips she might have used while pregnant. You should get advice from a person who has been through it, because you can benefit from their real-life experience.

187.   Start a journal or a pregnancy blog and post this online. Sharing your experiences can be very beneficial as the people who are reading your blog can offer you advice that is unique to your stage in

pregnancy. Also, this will give you documentation of how you felt during each step of the process.

188.   Get as much sleep as possible. When the baby arrives, it will be difficult for you to get the rest that you need, so it is important to find the time now to relax and de-stress. Extra sleep will also provide you with the energy that you need to stay active and maintain a baseline level of fitness leading up to your delivery.

189.   If you are pregnant with your first child, you should babysit for a friend with a young baby; this will give you an idea of what it is like to care for a newborn. Also, this will help to make you feel a little more comfortable once your baby is born.

190.   To help make sure the pregnancy is a healthy one, you should consider taking an HIV test. If you come up with a result that is positive, this will let the OB-GYN create a plan to help prevent spreading the disease to the baby. This also will help you attain help from medical professionals that know about HIV.

191.   Visit the dentist before you get pregnant. Studies have shown that periodontal disease can lead to inflammation; this inflammation has the potential to affect whether or not you develop preeclampsia.

Preeclampsia can have serious consequences for the health of both you and your child, so it is important to do everything you can to improve your teeth prior to conception.

192.   Writing down a birth plan will put your hopes, expectations and feelings about birth in perspective. You can outline exactly what you want to happen during the birth, easing your mind somewhat as you get closer to your due date. You can plan as many details as you want.

193.   Get your protein during pregnancy to ensure your baby's health growth. It is the material that structures every cell of your baby's growing body. If you are not taking in enough protein you are putting your baby at risk of issues with fetal growth. You should be taking in approximately 70 grams of protein a day while pregnant.

194.   You should definitely not be smoking while pregnant. If you smoke, the chances of many complications happening during the pregnancy go up. Smoking during pregnancy can cause many unfortunate events for both mother and baby. For you, ectopic pregnancy chances are significantly raised. Miscarriage or stillbirth is much more common when the mother smokes. You are also

putting your baby at risk for premature birth or birth defects.

195.   Make sure to be watching your weight when pregnant. Your doctor should tell you what you should be gaining (usually around 30 pounds), and you want to stick to that. Being severely overweight or underweight can cause health problems (diabetes) and birth defects (cleft palate) for your child. Being overweight can also cause a lot of health problems for you when pregnant.

196.   Know if you are HIV-positive or not. If you find out that you are, do not automatically freak out. HIV-positive women that are aware of this early on, have a higher chance of sparing their babies from getting this disease. You will want to make sure that you have an OB-GYN that is well educated about the care that will need to be taken and can explain all of your options for a safe pregnancy.

197.   Use a cold-water bath for swollen feet. One highly common symptom of pregnancy is swollen feet and ankles, especially in the heat. A cold water bath can reduce the blood flow to your feet, which in turn will reduce the inflammation. It also cools you down and gives you an excuse to be off your feet for a few minutes.

198.   Get some good maternity clothes whenever you require them. You will be more comfortable, and you will have more clothing that you can wear out of the house during your pregnancy. Don't be afraid to purchase maternity clothes early on. The only person who can determine what is comfortable and appropriate is you.

199.   See your dentist if you are pregnant and care for your teeth. There are a variety of dental issues which can arise at this time. Always brush your teeth at least twice per day, and don't forget to floss and use mouthwash. Do not delay in seeing your dentist if you experience any issues.

200.   If you smoke, being pregnant is the greatest reason you will ever have to stop smoking so find a way to do it now! As stressful as being pregnant may be, jeopardizing the health of your baby is a million times more stressful. This is a great opportunity to get medical help to quit and have the strongest motivating factor to keep you smoke-free.

201.   Gentle exercise when you are pregnant is a beneficial thing. This can reduce your chances of a miscarriage, how long you're in labor, along with helping you lose the weight easier after birth.

202.   Avoid any chemicals that could harm your baby. Many cleaning products have a strong smell and can be found in your home, your work and anywhere else you go. When you breath in these fumes, they can harm your child. Use products that are only made out of natural ingredients.

203.   Sleeping can become increasingly difficult as you get towards the end of your pregnancy. Find a great body pillow or maternity pillow that works for you. These are designed to give you the full body support that you need as you sleep. You will wake up less often and have less pain in the morning.

204.   As soon as you feel contractions, call your doctor or go to your hospital right away, even if you have had false labor pains before. You do not want to be in labor at home and give birth without having the proper medical care for you and your newborn child.

205.   Leg cramps happen a lot in the late stages of pregnancy. Stretching before bed can lessen the frequency and severity of the cramps. Drink water early in the day and take potassium supplements or eat bananas, too.

206.   During pregnancy, you should always ensure that your body is fully supported during sleep. Many

stores sell body pillows made especially for pregnancy. In case you do not own a pillow like this, a regular pillow can be used for support. Think about actually having a pillow that is under your stomach as well as another pillow for your knee to rest atop.

207.   Sleeping will become harder for you during your pregnancy. During the third trimester, sleep on your left side, this will provide you with the best blood flow to your fetus, uterus and kidneys. Remember, not to lay on your back.

208.   Learn how to do pelvic tilts and use them as you get into late pregnancy. They are a lifesaver for the back pain that will start as you get further along in your pregnancy. As an extra added benefit, they also help the baby work its way into an optimum birthing position.

209.   Pregnancy can intensify the sense of smell, making everyday odors nauseating. You can avoid becoming nauseated by simply carrying some lavender oil or lemon along with a handkerchief. When you are passing an odor that you find insulting you can smell the oil on the handkerchief.

210.   When you are pregnant, you will want to limit the amount of alcohol that you consume. This

means that when you are out with your friends, you will need to become more responsible for the sake of your baby. Practice good drinking habits to maximize the success of your pregnancy.

211.   Allow yourself to indulge in some of your cravings. You want to try and maintain a healthy diet during pregnancy, but it is okay to eat some unhealthy foods in moderation. Make sure to stay away from brie and feta cheese, herbal teas and raw sprouts, which could all negatively affect your baby's health.

212.   Be sure to find a good prenatal vitamin. In many cases your doctor will prescribe the best one for you but you can also find them over the counter. Be sure that it has at least 0.4 mg of folic acid in it. You may also want to look for an additional source of iron to take while you are pregnant.

213.   Make sure to get enough folic acid during your pregnancy. Folic acid is a major component to reducing the risk of neural defects like spina bifida. Lots of foods have been fortified with folic acid so keep an eye out for those on your shopping trips. Also make sure that your prenatal vitamins include folic acid.

214.   It is a good idea to pack your hospital bag when you reach 37 weeks or so. You are more likely to remember the items that you will both want and need while in the hospital if you aren't tossing things into a bag as you rush out the door.

215.   Stop smoking immediately if you have found out that you are pregnant or if are trying to become pregnant. Smoking, as we all know, is incredibly dangerous for us but it becomes even more important to quit when we are trying to take care of a new life. Talk with your doctor immediately if you are having trouble quitting.

216.   Remove any potentially harmful chemicals from your home. Cleaning solutions with harmful chemicals are a huge hazard in the home, so you might want to start using natural replacements. Once you have had the baby, make sure these chemicals are not in your home to ensure they don't cause any harm.

217.   Inform any doctor before a medical procedure if you are pregnant or planning on becoming pregnant. This includes your dentist as well. There are certain drugs that shouldn't be given and procedures that shouldn't be done for a women who is pregnant or on her way to pregnancy.

218.   Buy new shoes. As your pregnancy progresses, the extra weight will throw off your center of gravity, putting additional pressure on your feet. This can cause both fluid retention and flat feet. Purchase some comfortable shoes that give you good support; they will alleviate some of the previously mentioned concerns.

219.   If you are not sure how to handle a child or a newborn, talk to the mothers that you know. Offer to babysit for them. This way you are getting some experience, and your friend is getting a well deserved break from being a mother. Just keep in mind that no two children are the same!

220.   Invest in comfortable shoes when you're pregnant, as it will definitely help you. You are walking around with a lot of extra weight that your body is not use to, and it will take its tole on your feet. You will find they will start to swell, and you need shoes that are non-restrictive to battle this.

221.   When everyone around you wants you to eat when pregnant, find a way to say no. Although your caloric intake should somewhat increase, being pregnant isn't an excuse to pig out all the time. You have the right to make healthy food choices.

222.   Make sure the prescription drugs you are taking are not dangerous to the health of your baby. Every prescription drug on the market has a "pregnancy class" that tells you whether the drug is safe to take during pregnancy. If you are taking a drug that is unsafe for pregnant women, ask your doctor about alternatives. Most drugs have one or more.

223.   Don't start worrying if you aren't "showing" your pregnancy for a while. Most new moms don't start showing visible signs of pregnancy until they are in their 6th month. Subsequent pregnancies usually show earlier in the course of the pregnancy as the body has already been there and done that.

224.   Towards the end of the second trimester, massage your belly on a daily basis. Place a few pillows behind the back to ensure you aren't lying down flat, and sit yourself down on a bed or couch. Use oil as opposed to lotion while massaging your belly lightly. Play relaxing music and do not forget to breathe. Not only will your belly benefit, but your baby will be calmed as well.

225.   It is a good idea to pack your hospital bag when you reach 37 weeks or so. You are more likely to remember the items that you will both want and need while in the hospital if you aren't tossing things into a bag as you rush out the door.

226.   Always buy maternity clothes that are the correct size. Sometimes vanity keeps a woman from switching from their everyday clothes to maternity clothes. If you wear clothes that fit you, you will feel much better.

227.   Don't be afraid to say no to anything you don't want to do. If you are too tired to keep a movie date, it's okay to skip it. You need to make sure that you are taking care of your body the best that you can, and everyone who is close to you will respect this.

228.   Many people want to keep their pregnancy hidden from people for the first three months. It is better to choose one person that you can confide in. This will allow you to get release from everything that is going on in your life and talk about what is bothering you.

229.   One way to help to get rid of the back pain that sometimes occurs in late pregnancy is to practice pelvic tilts. Continuing to exercise in this way will not only help with the pain, it may also move your baby into a good birth position at the same time.

230.   Take breastfeeding classes or visit a La Leche Meeting before giving birth. These classes and

support groups can help you to prepare for the reality of breastfeeding a newborn, which can at times be stressful. They can also put you in contact with other pregnant woman and so, offer support through your pregnancy as well.

231. If you get diagnosed with gestational diabetes or some other issue that pertains to strictly the time when you are pregnant, know that this is just a temporary thing. It will help you get through the days of your pregnancy knowing that as soon as you are holding your baby you will know that it was all worth it.

232. Figure out what you want your birthing plan to be. Know that it does not have to be written out or formal if that is not your style. It is just so that you know what it is that you will want once you go into labor and can express it to the medical staff. Make sure your partner knows what your wishes are so he can speak for you in case you can not.

233. Take time every day to relax and enjoy yourself and your pregnancy. Pregnancy is a stressful time, and once the baby is born you will have much less time to yourself. Take advantage of the time now to relax, meditate, and reconnect with yourself and your unborn child. Your blood pressure will thank you.

234.   Adopt a healthier diet so your baby gets all the vitamin and nutrients it needs. If you had a habit of consuming a lot of fatty foods before becoming pregnant, you need to change your lifestyle quickly. Starting today, eat more vegetables, lean meats and fresh fruits.

235.   Get prenatal vitamins from your doctor or over the counter and make sure you take them on a regular basis. A good prenatal vitamin will take care of the needs of both you and your new baby. Make sure that your vitamin contains 0.4 mgs of folic acid for optimum brain development.

236.   Before you get pregnant you should read a book about being pregnant. This way you will know what to expect during pregnancy. Pregnancy books can also teach you many different things you may not have known about being pregnant. You will learn new things along with terminology about pregnancy.

237.   Hire a doula. This is a birth coach who can guide you through the process of pregnancy. She can give you support and ideas during your labor and delivery. They can offer experience and comfort and help guide you and your partner through the process.

238.   Keeping a food diary will help you to remember to eat well and keep up with all the vitamins that you need. You will also be able to see if you are not feeling well, that there may be some type of food you are eating that may be triggering that reaction.

239.   If you are pregnant, try to go swimming when you can. Not only is it a healthy exercise for all people, but for pregnant woman, it helps prevent those pesky leg aches and keeps you from gaining too much weight. Do not over do it though. If you feel yourself getting fatigued, stop.

240.   Don't eat or drink items with caffeine in them if you are pregnant. Caffeine can cause you not to get the rest you need and makes sleep less sound. Eating a few crackers can be an effective way to reduce nausea and allow you to sleep better. Your sleeping patterns are sure to benefit from a proper diet.

241.   If you have felt your baby moving around in your stomach, and then the movement stops for a few days, you should visit your doctor. Although this may mean nothing, there could be a problem with the baby that your doctor can help fix if taken care of in time.

242. If you find it hard to stick to a healthy diet during pregnancy, ask your partner to join you as you change your old eating habits to new healthy ones. It is always easier to make the right choices when you have a helpful partner to support you. Both of you will see the benefit of eating more vegetables, whole grains and fruit.

243. Avoid being seated in an immobile position for extended periods of time. Pregnancy can make an expectant mother's feet and ankles swell. This is most likely because of the significant increase of fluids in your body during pregnancy. A lot of the time, swelling is increased after sitting for awhile in a car or at a desk. There are several things you can do to help relieve the swelling. Try sleeping on the left side of your body, avoid tight socks and sit with your ankles uncrossed.

244. Get plenty of pregnancy before, during and after your pregnancy! Exercise lowers your rick of miscarrying, makes your pregnancy easier, results in fewer complications during labor and can even make your labor shorter. Regardless of whether you are already pregnant or you are trying to get pregnant, exercise makes an easier time of the whole experience.

245.   Some common foods can be dangerous to the unborn fetus. During your pregnancy, you should avoid anything that contains uncooked eggs like Caesar dressing, unpasteurized cheeses like queso blanco and under-cooked meats. Listeria can be present in precooked meats such as hot dogs and deli meats, so it is important to reheat them before consumption. For more information visit the CDC website or discuss the topic with your doctor.

246.   Reduce or remove the amount of caffeine and sugar in your diet to improve your sleep and overall health. Eating or drinking large amounts of caffeine and sugar are not good for your health or your baby's, plus they can significantly impact the amount and quality of sleep you get.

247.   Take a critical eye to the exercises you did before pregnancy to see if it is something it is safe for you to continue. Certain sports are no-brainers to avoid. Stay away from long distance running or running on steep inclines. Avoid things that involve rapid jerky movements like tennis or basketball.

248.   Ask your doctor to check your thyroid if you are considering becoming pregnant. Hypothyroidism is a fairly common disorder that can affect your ability to carry a baby to term. It can also cause learning disabilities in your unborn child. If you are already

pregnant, there is a simple, safe test that can be done to determine if you have an under-active metabolism.

249.   Stop smoking before you get pregnant. Smoking can affect your ability to conceive, so find something that will help you stop. You should talk to your doctor to see what recommendations they have to help you quit. There are many options available such as pills and patches.

250.   Talk to your friends and family, especially those that have been pregnant, or are currently pregnant. They will be able to support you and help you if you have any questions or if you need anything. Those who have been through it before can be some of the best resources you have.

251.   Engage in Kegel exercises each day. This activity can improve your pelvic muscles, which affect your bladder, bowels and uterus. Kegels will help with your delivery, and they can be done just about anywhere, including in the car or at work. To do them correctly, you should squeeze like you want to stop yourself from using the bathroom. Hold this position for three seconds and then relax for three. Do this in sets of ten.

252.   Be sure not to tend to cat litter when you are pregnant. You could get toxoplasmosis from changing a litter box. Felines can carry the parasite that causes toxoplasmosis. If a pregnant woman becomes infected and passes the infection to the fetus, a range of serious consequences can result, including birth defects, miscarriage, or even infant death.

253.   Once you have determined if you are having a boy or girl it is a good time to start decorating a room and picking out clothes. The more time you have before the baby actually arrives to prepare the better because the room will turn out nicer and you'll have more time to select better clothes.

254.   Leg cramps are a common issue for pregnant women. Stretching before bed can lessen the frequency and severity of the cramps. A high intake of fluids, particularly water, will also help keep cramps away, but make sure to drink water throughout the day, rather than right before bed, in order to prevent frequent wakings related to a full bladder.

255.   Increase your intake of cereals, asparagus, lentils, oranges and orange juice. These foods are all rich in folic acid, which helps the development of the baby's neural cord and creates red blood cells for

your unborn child. It is ideal to begin consuming these foods even before you start trying to conceive.

256.   Get your things together for your trip to the hospital when you're into your third trimester. You will not like the results if you procrastinate. You will want to include your birth plan, camera with extra batteries, and insurance cards.

257.   Make sure that you communicate with your partner (if you have one) about your feelings and your needs. You may know that you need to be touched or loved more often to feel supported, but they don't. You have to tell them what you need before you can expect to receive it.

258.   Stay away from anything that could harm you or your baby. This includes cigarettes, alcohol and even over-the-counter medications. Talk to your doctor about anything you are considering taking and let them advise you on the best course of action. All these substances could have a negative impact on your unborn child's development.

259.   When planning to become pregnant, see you doctor prior to conception. Once you have seen the doctor and have gotten cleared to conceive, start changing your eating habits to include a healthy

variety of foods. Start exercising now! It will help you stay in shape during the pregnancy and lower the risk of miscarriage.

260.   Put your birth plan in writing and share it with your doctor before you go into labor. Having your plan in writing helps you focus on the type of delivery you want and helps your doctor understand what you want. Even though unexpected events can result in changes, having your plan documented gives you peace of mind before going into labor.

261.   Talk to your employer as soon as you are comfortable about your pregnancy. Depending on your work environment, you may need to make arrangements for special equipment or changes in duties during your pregnancy. Giving your employer time to prepare reduces your stress and makes it more likely you can work throughout your pregnancy.

262.   Talk with your doctor before starting any exercise routine during pregnancy. There may be certain activities that you shouldn't do or some limitations they would like to put on how much you do. Write a plan of what you wanted to do and go over it with your doctor at your next appointment.

263.   You are pregnant, so now is the time to celebrate. You should avoid alcohol, of course, but you should not stop having some fun. You can make a toast to your little bundle of love with a glass of sparkling cider. You could even go all out, and have a party to announce your fantastic news. This is something to be celebrated!

264.   Tour a few birth facilities before delivering your baby. Hospital births are popular, but a birthing center might be more your style. Some facilities even offer practitioners who will perform home births. Touring several different types of birthing facilities will let you know the pros and cons of each, and help you to make an educated decision.

265.   For pregnant women, make sure that you stretch your legs, before going to sleep every night. This is because many pregnant women get intense muscle cramps while they are sleeping, which could be easily prevented, if they stretch. Spend about 5 minutes flexing all of your muscles, before even climbing into bed.

266.   A good thing to do when pregnant is to see your practitioner on a regular basis. This will not only help you in knowing about the things that pregnant people should know but it also will help you in

knowing how to have a healthy pregnancy. This act can help in having a very smooth pregnancy.

267.   A tip quite often given to pregnant women is to avoid heavy lifting. This is a tip that ought to be taken quite seriously. Anything can happen to the baby in the womb, and it is important not to do anything that might put the mother, or the child, in a dangerous situation.

268.   Learn how to read nutrition labels and find out what to avoid. Stay with items that are low in fat and low in calories. Keep stocked with items that are high in fiber. If you do have a sugary snack, drink it with a glass of milk to keep your blood sugar levels normal.

269.   Be sure to see your doctor before becoming pregnant. Not only does this help establish a healthy start to your prenatal care should you become pregnant, it also allows your doctor to check for any conditions that might require special care, or worse, discover conditions that would make pregnancy dangerous.

270.   Pregnancy can be a stressful time for couples. So it is better to work on relationship issues as they arise than waiting until after the baby arrives. Counseling can help couples communicate better

and strengthen your relationship, which in turn will help you both be better prepared to handle your new baby as partners.

271.   Be prepared for the hospital keep an old towel and a plastic bag in your car just in case your water breaks on the way to the hospital. Pack a robe for pacing the hospital halls, as well as nonskid slipper socks. Fill a small bag with electronics, such as an iPod for music and a still-photo and video camera. You will also need your insurance card, toiletries and a going home outfit for you and the baby. Staying prepared ensures this stressful time is easier, and keeps your emotions on a more even keel.

272.   Once you enter your third trimester, do a daily belly massage. You should place a few pillows behind you, and sit at a comfortable angle on the couch or your bed. Use light pressure and maybe oil, but never lotion when massaging your belly. Try to breathe and listen to some relaxing music. This keeps you calm and has positive effects on the baby.

273.   Before your child arrives, post a reminder to yourself in a prominent location in your home to add your baby to your health insurance plan. You usually have 30 days to do so after your child is born, but it is easy to forget during the haze of new parenthood. If delayed too long, this could leave

your child uninsured until annual enrollment season rolls around.

274.   If you experience symptoms like blurred vision, pain in your right side, frequent headaches, very rapid weight gain, or cola-colored urine in the second half of your pregnancy, report them to your doctor immediately. You may be developing preeclampsia, a pregnancy-related condition that can be life-threatening. Your doctor may need to perform tests to check for protein in your urine, and your blood pressure will be closely monitored.

275.   There are several ways to find childbirth classes to prepare you for the challenges of labor and delivery. Talking to friends who have just had a baby is one way to get a personal recommendation for a good class. You can also contact your hospital or health insurance provider for suggestions for classes open to you.

276.   When pregnant, never use salicylic acid for treating acne. It's proven to exfoliate skin and clean it deeply, but it's also known to harm unborn children in the womb. Use milder natural cleansers to treat acne during prenancy.

277.   Get your protein during pregnancy to ensure your baby's health growth. It is the material that

structures every cell of your baby's growing body. If you are not taking in enough protein you are putting your baby at risk of issues with fetal growth. You should be taking in approximately 70 grams of protein a day while pregnant.

278.   Consume at least 15 milligrams of zinc each day when you are pregnant. Many women have a zinc deficiency during pregnancy. This can affect their baby's growth and immune system. Some studies have indicated that not consuming enough zinc can also affect the immune system of your unborn child's offspring.

279.   Do not do too much when you are exercising while you are pregnant. This will ensure that you do not overextend yourself. It is very important to not hurt yourself when you are exercising when pregnant. It can not only make your pregnancy tougher on you but also on the baby, as well.

280.   If you have just discovered that you are pregnant, you will have to decide when to tell others. This decision is very personal and will be different for each person. One person will tell everybody on earth before her pregnancy test even turns positive. Another woman may be superstitious, and prefer to wait until she feels her

pregnancy is far enough along that she doesn't feel any problems will arise. Do what feels right to you.

281.   Hit up the bookstore or library and get books about pregnancy. Being armed with knowledge will help you deal with all the changes that your body will go through and teach you how to keep yourself healthy. Pregnancy is natural, but the more information you have about the process, the better it will go.

282.   Go ahead and give in to your pregnancy cravings. Doctors aren't quite sure if cravings are a result of emotional changes or of nutritional deficits in your diet, but not getting the foods you crave can be stressful during a time when you don't need the added stress. Just be careful that your diet is healthy overall.

283.   Keep exercising. Especially in those first few months when you may not feel so great, it is even more important to discipline yourself to staying active. Go for a walk in the morning or the evening. Do some light weight lifting. This will keep you body toned during pregnancy and make losing weight after the birth much easier.

284.   One of the very basic things that pregnant women should do in order to achieve a healthy

pregnancy is to start changing the food habits that they have. It is very important to have a healthy variety of foods in order to properly nourish the baby.

285.   Read a pregnancy book. They provide expectant parents with a wealth of information on what to expect both during the pregnancy and after the baby is born. They give new parents piece of mind by helping them plan, and they answer questions that they may not want to ask their friends or family members.

286.   When you are pregnant, it's recommended that you be checked for any sexually transmitted diseases. These diseases, if left untreated, can cause serious health issues for both you and the baby. There are a wide variety of tests that can be taken to check for these diseases. Some may require that you consider delivery by Caesarian section

287.   Your legs may cramp during your last trimester. Stretching at bedtime will help with this. Drinking plenty of water and making sure you're getting enough potassium in your diet can also help you avoid cramps,

288.   Listen to soft music and take a hot shower before bed time. Sleep can become more difficult

the further along that you get. Avoid sleep aids and other pills by putting your body and your mind into a restful state before you even get into bed. A hot shower and soothing music will do this for you.

289.   Do not let stretch marks stress you out, as they are completely unavoidable for many women. While applying cocoa butter and other creams may help to lessen the itching and irritation that comes along with rapid stretching of the skin, they cannot do much to prevent the marks themselves.

290.   When you are pregnant, one of the things that you will want to stop as soon as possible is smoking. Smoking can cause birth defects for your baby, so stopping immediately will limit this risk. Join support groups to increase the willpower that you will need to stop this unhealthy habit. You must also insist that people who smoke do not do so in the same room as you.

291.   Take some precautions when traveling by plane. The second trimester is often noted as the best time to fly, because you are not experiencing morning sickness as often, and there is less risk of miscarriage. Always speak to your doctor first and make sure to drink a lot of water on the plane to stay hydrated. Get up and walk frequently to help avoid blood clots.

292.   When trying to perform kick counts late in pregnancy, your previously active baby may occasionally scare you with fewer movements than normal. If you are concerned, try drinking a caffeinated soda or something with a bit of sugar in it. Often, this is enough to wake up your baby and jump-start his or her movements again.

293.   Visit the dentist before you get pregnant. Studies have shown that periodontal disease can lead to inflammation; this inflammation has the potential to affect whether or not you develop preeclampsia. Preeclampsia can have serious consequences for the health of both you and your child, so it is important to do everything you can to improve your teeth prior to conception.

294.   Belching, gas, and heartburn are all side effects of being pregnant. To help deal with these types of issues during your pregnancy, you should stay upright after you eat, stay away from offending foods, and drink a glass of milk with honey; these are all ways to help you minimize some of the gas and heartburn.

295.   Find a good position for sleeping. During your third trimester, sleeping on your left side will put you in the best position for your blood flow to

reach the fetus, your uterus and your kidneys. If you are more comfortable sleeping in a different position, that's okay, just make sure not to sleep on your back.

296.   It is best to avoid the use of salicylic acid for acne during your pregnancy. Although it may help your skin with it deep cleaning and exfoliating properties, it can harm your unborn child. To help control your acne and prevent breakouts while pregnant, use a mild daily cleanser.

297.   You should start taking a prenatal vitamin now. Taking a prenatal vitamin is great for your health. Prenatal vitamins can also help you conceive a baby. They are great for many different reasons and your doctor can help you find out which one is the best while trying to conceive.

298.   Make sure you are educated about pregnancy. There are so many books and websites that you can read that will help you out. If you know what is supposed to be going on, it will calm your nerves, and you will also be able to tell if something is wrong.

299.   Being sleepy in the first trimester is very normal. Your energy level will probably plummet as that baby is growing in leaps and bounds. Make sure that

you get lots of extra rest. Go to bed early and if you can change your schedule, wake up later. Don't be afraid to take a nap in the middle of the day either if you need it.

300.   Try not to wear clothing that is too tight when pregnant. This kind of clothing can actually cause your fetus to not get enough oxygen and make you uncomfortable. There are maternity jeans available for pregnant women. Also, when at home, try to wear sweatpants or pajama bottoms with a loose T-shirt.

301.   Pay a visit to the facility in which you plan to give birth. Look around and get a tour so you can meet the staff. Any questions you have can be answered and you may feel more calm. The dad in this situation can get his questions answered too, since it will most likely be them who are speaking with the staff when you're in labor.

302.   Walk as much as you can when you've exceeded your due date and you want to go into labor. Walking helps naturally lower your baby to the ideal position for childbirth. Ask a partner to come along with you. Avoid dangerous techniques, such as contact exercising.

303.   Take a child birthing class. These classes will help you near the end of your pregnancy. They will teach you exactly what to expect, and your partner should go along to. You will probably watch a movie of someone giving birth, learn a lot of new breathing exercises, and probably meet some new friends too.

304.   When pregnant, avoid reclining after a meal. This can help your prevent heartburn. If you experience heartburn, you should sleep with your head elevated by pillows. Try to avoid foods that are spicy, acidic, or fried. These can be the main causes for heartburn during pregnancy. Those types of foods can also worsen your heartburn.

305.   When pregnant, you should exercise regularly. Exercising regularly throughout your pregnancy will help you avoid gaining excessive weight. Exercising can also increase your circulation which will help you prevent leg cramps at night. Try to avoid exercising in the evening as it will make it difficult for you to go to sleep.

306.   Eat plenty of fruit during your pregnancy. Many women get a boost of energy during the day from caffeine products; since these are not recommended during pregnancy, try fruit instead. People who consume bananas and apples, often notice an

increase in their energy levels. This comes from the natural sugars that these fruits contain.

307.   Try not drive alone during the later stages of your pregnancy, just in case you were to go into labor. Being alone in your car when you water breaks can mean you will be yourself when you deliver. This could cause your baby to be born improperly and can cause health problems for you.

308.   When you are pregnant, it is best to avoid or limit your caffeine intake. You can still have one cup of coffee in the morning, but no more than that. Try drinking decaff or half-caff if you can. Any caffeine that you drink will go straight to your baby and may have negative effects.

309.   Although it can be fun, when decorating your baby's nursery avoid painting or putting up wallpaper while you are pregnant to avoid the harmful fumes. Have your partner or some friends to take care of those jobs, and stay out of the room until the paint or wallpaper glue dries and the room is fume-free.

310.   When you want to conceive, it is a good idea to pay attention to your cycle. Then you'll be able to determine the best time for conception. You can learn how to tell if you skip a period and also if you

should try a pregnancy test at home to find out if you're pregnant.

311.   A healthy diet during pregnancy includes foods that are packed with nutrition to help your baby get off to a great start. Include a variety of foods that provide the fiber, vitamins and minerals that will help your baby develop properly. Get rid of the nutritionally empty junk foods that use up your daily calorie intake with no benefit to your baby.

312.   The most important thing to do during pregnancy is to look after yourself. If your body says it is tired, then sleep if you can. There is no point trying to maintain high standards of home tidiness if you are going to be exhausted for nine months and not enjoying the pregnancy. Remember to give yourself a break and take as much time out for yourself as needed.

www.ingramcontent.com/pod-product-compliance
Lightning Source LLC
Chambersburg PA
CBHW060747260726
48660CB00002B/518